THIS BOOK BELONGS TO:

CONTACT INFORMATION	
NAME:	
ADDRESS:	
PHONE:	

START / END DATES

_____ / _____ / _____   TO   _____ / _____ / _____

DEDICATION

This Cannabis Growers Journal is dedicated to all the weed enthusiasts out there who want to record all their marijuana growing adventures and document their findings in the process.

You are my inspiration for producing books and I'm honored to be a part of keeping all of your marijuana notes and records organized.

This journal notebook will help you record the details of your weed growing adventures.

Thoughtfully put together with these sections to record: Strain Name, Date Started, Seed or Clone, Indica, Hybrid or Stavia, Feminized or Autoflower, Plant Count, Date Harvested, Date Begin & End Cure, Aroma, Bud Density, & more.

HOW TO USE THIS BOOK

The purpose of this book is to keep all of your Marijuana Harvesting notes all in one place. It will help keep you organized.

This Cannabis Growers Journal will allow you to accurately document every detail about your weed growing adventures.

Here are examples of the prompts for you to fill in and write about your experience in this book:

1. Strain Name
2. Date Started
3. Seed or Clone
4. Indica, Hybrid, or Stavia
5. Feminized or Autoflower
6. Plant Count
7. Date Harvested
8. Date Begin & End Cure
9. Aroma
10. Bud Density
11. Trichome Color
12. Appearance
13. Notes
14. Feeding Schedule & Times

GROWERS JOURNAL

STRAIN NAME	
DATE STARTED	☐ SEED ☐ CLONE

INDICA   HYBRID   SATIVA

☐ FEMINIZED	☐ AUTOFLOWER	PLANT COUNT:	

DATE HARVESTED	DATE BEGIN CURE	DATE END CURE

AROMA

BUD DENSITY	TRICHOME COLOR
LOOSE 50% DENSE	WHITE 50% AMBER

APPEARANCE

ADDITIONAL NOTES

FEEDING SCHEDULE

WEEK #	☐ MILLILITER ☐ TABLESPOON ☐ TEASPOON				
	1	2	3	4	5
GROWTH STAGE					
PPM RANGE					

NOTES

RESERVOIR/BUCKET SIZE:				OPTIMAL PH:		
6	7	8	9	10	11	12

NOTES

GROWERS JOURNAL

STRAIN NAME	
DATE STARTED	☐ SEED ☐ CLONE

INDICA   HYBRID   SATIVA

☐ FEMINIZED	☐ AUTOFLOWER	PLANT COUNT:	

DATE HARVESTED	DATE BEGIN CURE	DATE END CURE

AROMA

BUD DENSITY

LOOSE   50%   DENSE

TRICHOME COLOR

WHITE   50%   AMBER

APPEARANCE

FEEDING SCHEDULE

WEEK #	☐ MILLILITER	☐ TABLESPOON	☐ TEASPOON		
	1	2	3	4	5
GROWTH STAGE					
PPM RANGE					

NOTES

RESERVOIR/BUCKET SIZE:				OPTIMAL PH:		
6	7	8	9	10	11	12

NOTES

GROWERS JOURNAL

STRAIN NAME	
DATE STARTED	☐ SEED ☐ CLONE

INDICA   HYBRID   SATIVA

☐ FEMINIZED	☐ AUTOFLOWER	PLANT COUNT:

DATE HARVESTED	DATE BEGIN CURE	DATE END CURE

AROMA

BUD DENSITY	TRICHOME COLOR
LOOSE 50% DENSE	WHITE 50% AMBER

APPEARANCE

FEEDING SCHEDULE

WEEK #	☐ MILLILITER	☐ TABLESPOON	☐ TEASPOON		
	1	2	3	4	5
GROWTH STAGE					
PPM RANGE					

NOTES

RESERVOIR/BUCKET SIZE:				OPTIMAL PH:		
6	7	8	9	10	11	12

NOTES

GROWERS JOURNAL

STRAIN NAME		
DATE STARTED		☐ SEED ☐ CLONE

INDICA   HYBRID   SATIVA

☐ FEMINIZED	☐ AUTOFLOWER	PLANT COUNT:	

DATE HARVESTED	DATE BEGIN CURE	DATE END CURE

AROMA

BUD DENSITY	TRICHOME COLOR
LOOSE 50% DENSE	WHITE 50% AMBER

APPEARANCE

FEEDING SCHEDULE

WEEK #	☐ MILLILITER ☐ TABLESPOON ☐ TEASPOON				
	1	2	3	4	5
GROWTH STAGE					
PPM RANGE					

NOTES

RESERVOIR/BUCKET SIZE:				OPTIMAL PH:		
6	7	8	9	10	11	12

NOTES

GROWERS JOURNAL

STRAIN NAME	
DATE STARTED	☐ SEED ☐ CLONE

INDICA   HYBRID   SATIVA

☐ FEMINIZED	☐ AUTOFLOWER	PLANT COUNT:	

DATE HARVESTED	DATE BEGIN CURE	DATE END CURE

AROMA

BUD DENSITY	TRICHOME COLOR
LOOSE 50% DENSE	WHITE 50% AMBER

APPEARANCE

FEEDING SCHEDULE

WEEK #	☐ MILLILITER	☐ TABLESPOON	☐ TEASPOON		
	1	2	3	4	5
GROWTH STAGE					
PPM RANGE					

NOTES

RESERVOIR/BUCKET SIZE:				OPTIMAL PH:		
6	7	8	9	10	11	12

NOTES

GROWERS JOURNAL

STRAIN NAME	
DATE STARTED	☐ SEED ☐ CLONE

INDICA   HYBRID   SATIVA

☐ FEMINIZED	☐ AUTOFLOWER	PLANT COUNT:	

DATE HARVESTED	DATE BEGIN CURE	DATE END CURE

AROMA

BUD DENSITY

LOOSE   50%   DENSE

TRICHOME COLOR

WHITE   50%   AMBER

APPEARANCE

FEEDING SCHEDULE

WEEK #	☐ MILLILITER	☐ TABLESPOON	☐ TEASPOON		
	1	2	3	4	5
GROWTH STAGE					
PPM RANGE					

NOTES

RESERVOIR/BUCKET SIZE:				OPTIMAL PH:		
6	7	8	9	10	11	12

NOTES

GROWERS JOURNAL

STRAIN NAME	
DATE STARTED	☐ SEED ☐ CLONE

INDICA   HYBRID   SATIVA

☐ FEMINIZED	☐ AUTOFLOWER	PLANT COUNT:

DATE HARVESTED	DATE BEGIN CURE	DATE END CURE

AROMA

BUD DENSITY

LOOSE   50%   DENSE

TRICHOME COLOR

WHITE   50%   AMBER

APPEARANCE

ADDITIONAL NOTES

FEEDING SCHEDULE

	☐ MILLILITER	☐ TABLESPOON	☐ TEASPOON		
WEEK #	1	2	3	4	5
GROWTH STAGE					
PPM RANGE					

NOTES

RESERVOIR/BUCKET SIZE:				OPTIMAL PH:		
6	7	8	9	10	11	12

NOTES

GROWERS JOURNAL

STRAIN NAME	
DATE STARTED	☐ SEED ☐ CLONE

INDICA   HYBRID   SATIVA

☐ FEMINIZED	☐ AUTOFLOWER	PLANT COUNT:

DATE HARVESTED	DATE BEGIN CURE	DATE END CURE

AROMA

BUD DENSITY

LOOSE   50%   DENSE

TRICHOME COLOR

WHITE   50%   AMBER

APPEARANCE

ADDITIONAL NOTES

FEEDING SCHEDULE

WEEK #	☐ MILLILITER	☐ TABLESPOON	☐ TEASPOON		
	1	2	3	4	5
GROWTH STAGE					
PPM RANGE					

NOTES

RESERVOIR/BUCKET SIZE: | | | | OPTIMAL PH: | |

6	7	8	9	10	11	12

NOTES

GROWERS JOURNAL

STRAIN NAME	
DATE STARTED	☐ SEED ☐ CLONE

INDICA   HYBRID   SATIVA

☐ FEMINIZED	☐ AUTOFLOWER	PLANT COUNT:	

DATE HARVESTED	DATE BEGIN CURE	DATE END CURE

AROMA

BUD DENSITY	TRICHOME COLOR
LOOSE 50% DENSE	WHITE 50% AMBER

APPEARANCE

FEEDING SCHEDULE

	☐ MILLILITER	☐ TABLESPOON	☐ TEASPOON		
WEEK #	1	2	3	4	5
GROWTH STAGE					
PPM RANGE					

NOTES

RESERVOIR/BUCKET SIZE:

OPTIMAL PH:

6	7	8	9	10	11	12

NOTES

GROWERS JOURNAL

STRAIN NAME	
DATE STARTED	☐ SEED ☐ CLONE

INDICA   HYBRID   SATIVA

☐ FEMINIZED	☐ AUTOFLOWER	PLANT COUNT:	

DATE HARVESTED	DATE BEGIN CURE	DATE END CURE

AROMA

BUD DENSITY	TRICHOME COLOR
LOOSE 50% DENSE	WHITE 50% AMBER

APPEARANCE

ADDITIONAL NOTES

FEEDING SCHEDULE

WEEK #	☐ MILLILITER	☐ TABLESPOON	☐ TEASPOON		
	1	2	3	4	5
GROWTH STAGE					
PPM RANGE					

NOTES

RESERVOIR/BUCKET SIZE:				OPTIMAL PH:		
6	7	8	9	10	11	12

NOTES

GROWERS JOURNAL

STRAIN NAME	
DATE STARTED	☐ SEED ☐ CLONE

INDICA HYBRID SATIVA

☐ FEMINIZED	☐ AUTOFLOWER	PLANT COUNT:	

DATE HARVESTED	DATE BEGIN CURE	DATE END CURE

AROMA

BUD DENSITY	TRICHOME COLOR
LOOSE 50% DENSE	WHITE 50% AMBER

APPEARANCE

FEEDING SCHEDULE

WEEK #	☐ MILLILITER	☐ TABLESPOON	☐ TEASPOON		
	1	2	3	4	5
GROWTH STAGE					
PPM RANGE					

NOTES

RESERVOIR/BUCKET SIZE: OPTIMAL PH:

6	7	8	9	10	11	12

NOTES

GROWERS JOURNAL

STRAIN NAME		
DATE STARTED		☐ SEED ☐ CLONE

INDICA   HYBRID   SATIVA

| ☐ FEMINIZED | ☐ AUTOFLOWER | PLANT COUNT: | |

DATE HARVESTED	DATE BEGIN CURE	DATE END CURE

AROMA

BUD DENSITY	TRICHOME COLOR
LOOSE 50% DENSE	WHITE 50% AMBER

APPEARANCE

FEEDING SCHEDULE

WEEK #	☐ MILLILITER	☐ TABLESPOON	☐ TEASPOON		
	1	2	3	4	5
GROWTH STAGE					
PPM RANGE					

NOTES

RESERVOIR/BUCKET SIZE:				OPTIMAL PH:		
6	7	8	9	10	11	12

NOTES

GROWERS JOURNAL

STRAIN NAME	
DATE STARTED	☐ SEED ☐ CLONE

INDICA   HYBRID   SATIVA

☐ FEMINIZED	☐ AUTOFLOWER	PLANT COUNT:	

DATE HARVESTED	DATE BEGIN CURE	DATE END CURE

AROMA

BUD DENSITY	TRICHOME COLOR
LOOSE 50% DENSE	WHITE 50% AMBER

APPEARANCE

FEEDING SCHEDULE

WEEK #	☐ MILLILITER	☐ TABLESPOON	☐ TEASPOON		
	1	2	3	4	5
GROWTH STAGE					
PPM RANGE					

NOTES

RESERVOIR/BUCKET SIZE:				OPTIMAL PH:		
6	7	8	9	10	11	12

NOTES

GROWERS JOURNAL

STRAIN NAME	
DATE STARTED	☐ SEED ☐ CLONE

INDICA   HYBRID   SATIVA

☐ FEMINIZED	☐ AUTOFLOWER	PLANT COUNT:	

DATE HARVESTED	DATE BEGIN CURE	DATE END CURE

AROMA

BUD DENSITY	TRICHOME COLOR
LOOSE 50% DENSE	WHITE 50% AMBER

APPEARANCE

ADDITIONAL NOTES

FEEDING SCHEDULE

	☐ MILLILITER	☑ TABLESPOON	☐ TEASPOON		
WEEK #	1	2	3	4	5
GROWTH STAGE					
PPM RANGE					

NOTES

RESERVOIR/BUCKET SIZE:				OPTIMAL PH:		
6	7	8	9	10	11	12

NOTES

GROWERS JOURNAL

STRAIN NAME	
DATE STARTED	☐ SEED ☐ CLONE

INDICA   HYBRID   SATIVA

☐ FEMINIZED	☐ AUTOFLOWER	PLANT COUNT:

DATE HARVESTED	DATE BEGIN CURE	DATE END CURE

AROMA

BUD DENSITY	TRICHOME COLOR
LOOSE 50% DENSE	WHITE 50% AMBER

APPEARANCE

FEEDING SCHEDULE

WEEK #	☐ MILLILITER	☐ TABLESPOON	☐ TEASPOON		
	1	2	3	4	5
GROWTH STAGE					
PPM RANGE					

NOTES

RESERVOIR/BUCKET SIZE:				OPTIMAL PH:		
6	7	8	9	10	11	12

NOTES

GROWERS JOURNAL

STRAIN NAME	
DATE STARTED	☐ SEED ☐ CLONE

INDICA   HYBRID   SATIVA

☐ FEMINIZED	☐ AUTOFLOWER	PLANT COUNT:	

DATE HARVESTED	DATE BEGIN CURE	DATE END CURE

AROMA

BUD DENSITY	TRICHOME COLOR
LOOSE 50% DENSE	WHITE 50% AMBER

APPEARANCE

ADDITIONAL NOTES

FEEDING SCHEDULE

WEEK #	☐ MILLILITER	☐ TABLESPOON	☐ TEASPOON		
	1	2	3	4	5
GROWTH STAGE					
PPM RANGE					

NOTES

RESERVOIR/BUCKET SIZE:				OPTIMAL PH:		
6	7	8	9	10	11	12

NOTES

GROWERS JOURNAL

STRAIN NAME	
DATE STARTED	☐ SEED ☐ CLONE

INDICA   HYBRID   SATIVA

☐ FEMINIZED	☐ AUTOFLOWER	PLANT COUNT:	

DATE HARVESTED	DATE BEGIN CURE	DATE END CURE

AROMA

BUD DENSITY	TRICHOME COLOR
LOOSE 50% DENSE	WHITE 50% AMBER

APPEARANCE

ADDITIONAL NOTES

FEEDING SCHEDULE

WEEK #	□ MILLILITER	□ TABLESPOON	□ TEASPOON		
	1	2	3	4	5
GROWTH STAGE					
PPM RANGE					

NOTES

RESERVOIR/BUCKET SIZE:				OPTIMAL PH:		
6	7	8	9	10	11	12

NOTES

GROWERS JOURNAL

STRAIN NAME	
DATE STARTED	☐ SEED ☐ CLONE

INDICA   HYBRID   SATIVA

☐ FEMINIZED	☐ AUTOFLOWER	PLANT COUNT:

DATE HARVESTED	DATE BEGIN CURE	DATE END CURE

AROMA

BUD DENSITY

LOOSE   50%   DENSE

TRICHOME COLOR

WHITE   50%   AMBER

APPEARANCE

FEEDING SCHEDULE

WEEK #	□ MILLILITER	□ TABLESPOON	□ TEASPOON		
	1	2	3	4	5
GROWTH STAGE					
PPM RANGE					

NOTES

RESERVOIR/BUCKET SIZE:				OPTIMAL PH:		
6	7	8	9	10	11	12

NOTES

GROWERS JOURNAL

STRAIN NAME	
DATE STARTED	☐ SEED ☐ CLONE

INDICA   HYBRID   SATIVA

☐ FEMINIZED	☐ AUTOFLOWER	PLANT COUNT:	

DATE HARVESTED	DATE BEGIN CURE	DATE END CURE

AROMA

BUD DENSITY	TRICHOME COLOR
LOOSE 50% DENSE	WHITE 50% AMBER

APPEARANCE

ADDITIONAL NOTES

FEEDING SCHEDULE

WEEK #	☐ MILLILITER	☐ TABLESPOON	☐ TEASPOON		
	1	2	3	4	5
GROWTH STAGE					
PPM RANGE					

NOTES

RESERVOIR/BUCKET SIZE:				OPTIMAL PH:		
6	7	8	9	10	11	12

NOTES

GROWERS JOURNAL

STRAIN NAME	
DATE STARTED	☐ SEED ☐ CLONE

INDICA   HYBRID   SATIVA

☐ FEMINIZED	☐ AUTOFLOWER	PLANT COUNT:	

DATE HARVESTED	DATE BEGIN CURE	DATE END CURE

AROMA

BUD DENSITY	TRICHOME COLOR
LOOSE 50% DENSE	WHITE 50% AMBER

APPEARANCE

ADDITIONAL NOTES

FEEDING SCHEDULE

	☐ MILLILITER	☐ TABLESPOON	☐ TEASPOON		
WEEK #	1	2	3	4	5
GROWTH STAGE					
PPM RANGE					

NOTES

RESERVOIR/BUCKET SIZE:				OPTIMAL PH:		
6	7	8	9	10	11	12

NOTES

GROWERS JOURNAL

STRAIN NAME	
DATE STARTED	☐ SEED ☐ CLONE

INDICA   HYBRID   SATIVA

☐ FEMINIZED	☐ AUTOFLOWER	PLANT COUNT:	

DATE HARVESTED	DATE BEGIN CURE	DATE END CURE

AROMA

BUD DENSITY

LOOSE   50%   DENSE

TRICHOME COLOR

WHITE   50%   AMBER

APPEARANCE

FEEDING SCHEDULE

WEEK #	☐ MILLILITER	☐ TABLESPOON	☐ TEASPOON		
	1	2	3	4	5
GROWTH STAGE					
PPM RANGE					

NOTES

RESERVOIR/BUCKET SIZE:				OPTIMAL PH:		
6	7	8	9	10	11	12

NOTES

GROWERS JOURNAL

STRAIN NAME	
DATE STARTED		☐ SEED ☐ CLONE

INDICA   HYBRID   SATIVA

| ☐ FEMINIZED | ☐ AUTOFLOWER | PLANT COUNT: | |

DATE HARVESTED	DATE BEGIN CURE	DATE END CURE

AROMA

BUD DENSITY

LOOSE   50%   DENSE

TRICHOME COLOR

WHITE   50%   AMBER

APPEARANCE

ADDITIONAL NOTES

FEEDING SCHEDULE

	☐ MILLILITER ☐ TABLESPOON ☐ TEASPOON				
WEEK #	1	2	3	4	5
GROWTH STAGE					
PPM RANGE					

NOTES

RESERVOIR/BUCKET SIZE:				OPTIMAL PH:		
6	7	8	9	10	11	12

NOTES

GROWERS JOURNAL

STRAIN NAME		
DATE STARTED		☐ SEED ☐ CLONE

INDICA   HYBRID   SATIVA

☐ FEMINIZED	☐ AUTOFLOWER	PLANT COUNT:

DATE HARVESTED	DATE BEGIN CURE	DATE END CURE

AROMA

BUD DENSITY

LOOSE   50%   DENSE

TRICHOME COLOR

WHITE   50%   AMBER

APPEARANCE

FEEDING SCHEDULE

WEEK #	☐ MILLILITER	☐ TABLESPOON	☐ TEASPOON		
	1	2	3	4	5
GROWTH STAGE					
PPM RANGE					

NOTES

RESERVOIR/BUCKET SIZE:				OPTIMAL PH:		
6	7	8	9	10	11	12

NOTES

GROWERS JOURNAL

STRAIN NAME	
DATE STARTED	☐ SEED ☐ CLONE

INDICA   HYBRID   SATIVA

☐ FEMINIZED	☐ AUTOFLOWER	PLANT COUNT:

DATE HARVESTED	DATE BEGIN CURE	DATE END CURE

AROMA

BUD DENSITY

LOOSE   50%   DENSE

TRICHOME COLOR

WHITE   50%   AMBER

APPEARANCE

FEEDING SCHEDULE

WEEK #	☐ MILLILITER ☐ TABLESPOON ☐ TEASPOON				
	1	2	3	4	5
GROWTH STAGE					
PPM RANGE					

NOTES

RESERVOIR/BUCKET SIZE:				OPTIMAL PH:		
6	7	8	9	10	11	12

NOTES

Printed in the USA
CPSIA information can be obtained
at www.ICGtesting.com
LVHW020208260923
759348LV00013B/411